JOURNEY

OF

I0100177

DISCOVERY

Rosemary Argente

Journey of Discovery © Copyright Rosemary Argente

First edition 2017

Editor: Venus Alae-Carew

Cover: Kacha Walo at 2 months
Photos restored by Brian Sherman

Publishers: Asaina Books
Website: www.asainabooks.co.uk
Email: rosa@asainabooks.co.uk

Books by the same author:

Blantyre and Yawo Women
The Veil
The Promised Land – Companion to The Veil
Praying Mantis
Broken Temple
Praying Mantis
Difference
Share the Ride
Home From Home
Essays and Poetry
The Place Beyond
Caesar and Mapanga Homestead

Novels:
All Mine to Have
Farewell Sophomore
The Stream of Memory
A British Throne Scandal

Science Fiction:
Farewell to the Aeroplane

Booklets:
Journey of Discovery
Enduring Fountain – Health and Well-being
Katherine of the Wheel
Cooking With Asaina

ACKNOWLEDGEMENTS

Thanks to Lorna Argente for granting permission to write a booklet about her journey to and discovery of planet Earth. Thanks also to Chris McCoy for his excerpt from "*Listen – A Baby's Thoughts*"

Every conception
As every birth is a winner
-    Author

1

BABY'S JOURNEY began before she was born. First she had to win the sperm race. Along with her fellow spermatozoon; with lashing tails; tips empowered by chromosome energy; void of limbs, but agile; all are accomplished swimmers – heading for the fertilisation point: the ovum (see postscript).

****

IT WAS A THURSDAY NIGHT when Mami's labour pains began. She was taken to Dr Antao's house where he delivered babies. On the second morning after, like the moment the universe was created, Baby entered the world by a vibrant cry, handicapped, helpless, no limb to touch, or bipedal, gasping for air, no speech to communicate with. Pain from the sudden egress, anger or fright at separation from the protection of the womb, or charged with like velocity to the fertilising point at conception? God's overall embrace, *an overwhelming intake of air*, the God surrounding us in the very air we breathe. She was born healthy, and perfect in every way.   -

The first on the scene was baby's father. In those days fathers were not permitted to be present at baby's birth.

"She is beautiful! he exclaimed with great joy.

"Well, she has to be, both her parents are beautiful", says the doctor's wife.

Perhaps no one was more proud than Anganga, the great grand-mother, when she said to Baby's mother:

"Have you reached this milestone?   You now have the knowledge and the experience on what it takes to bring a human being into the world! You have made it!"

****

Baby tired, continues in a gentle cry. Then, when all is settled, little Baby's eyes focus on people and things around her, trying to understand the world she has entered into, even at the minim of birth just passed. At birth awareness combines the other part of her perception which is two-dimensional: the classification of the natural world, one's perception of natural surroundings such as the earth, sky, light of day, dark of night, atmosphere, space, surface of the ground and others. The other aspect is the social conditioning of the cultural world. From the moment of birth the infant's mind will absorb, by watching and mimicking.

'Cry' in varying degrees, is all the speech she has to indicate discomfort or her momentous needs. She is best at peace and contentment when she is feeding at the breast. Baby is all awareness as her eyes were moving around the room and focusing on people present:

> *"Listening, listening to a cacophony of noise. There were children squealing, laughing and shouting. Men were telling jokes as they sharpened tools and mended nets. Women were carrying water and chatting, passing on the latest gossip. The crackle of burning firewood, the hiss of steam from the cooking pots, the noise of everyday life. The birds were calling, animals in the distance grunting and growling. The wind rustled through the branches of*

4

the trees. There were soft words of encouragement from my mother as she put her nipple to my mouth. The repeated sucking sound as her milk found its way to my stomach. All this I heard, less than one day old. Although I was aware, I did not understand what all the strange sounds meant."

****

On the following Monday morning the sound of a tune from a guitar wafted into the maternity room.

"Where is that coming from?" Baby's Mami asked.

"He must be a loafer, playing a guitar on a Monday morning when he should be out looking for a job!" The midwife replied.

"It must be a good sign. He is serenading Baby."

Gani, Grandmother nick names her Kacha Walo. We never came to know what it meant but it was a phrase formed by a loving heart.

****

Baby's daddy always sung her a lullaby:

 Good night, little girlie goodnight,

 Close your eyes its time to go to sleep.

 A bed time story though I could tell,

 I'd rather play the banjo than croon a lullaby.

 Some day you'll go your way,

5

It may not be an easy one.

Don't give in, try your best to win.

Good night little girlie goodnight.

About half way through the lullaby Kacha Walo disappeared into dreamland...

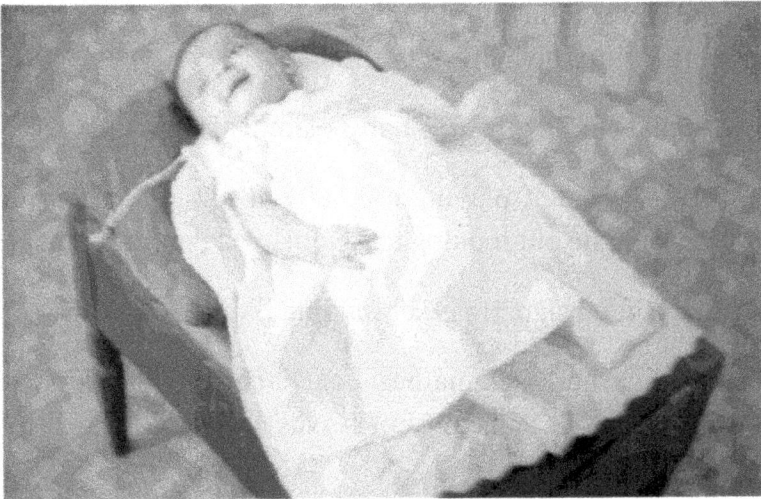

At two months

Mimicking Govindram -

Mami takes Kacha to Blantyre for shopping. It was the first time it became evident that at two months Kacha was mimicking the actions of people around her. They go into Bombay Bazaar and Mami talks to Govindaram, owner of the shop. He has a habit of wringing his hands when talking and Kacha Walo is trying hard to mimic him. Her whole face contorted, with her lips rolled as if she was going to whistle while manipulating her hands together.

ANGANGA (great grand mother) could make Kacha Walo laugh as early as four weeks old, but the after effect of laughing was hiccups and that frightened Mami. It is not until she is two months old that she responds, by smiling, to mother's "Chiki! Chiki!" Attempt at conversation.

Rex, faithful dog -

Mami took a dog and named him Rex. He was a mongrel mixture of ridgeback and Labrador Retriever. He was so loyal and was always at Baby's side, protecting her twenty-four hours a day. Wherever Kacha went Rex followed beside her pram.

Atowe injowe -

Kacha then begins to form vocabulary. She carried the "Atowe. Injowe" for several weeks, whenever she wanted to express something, only understood by Mami. Until she formed more advanced vocabulary.

We visit Lillian, the friend, who gives Kacha an apple. Lillian had been filing her nails and was holding the steel nail file. Kacha kept demanding saying:

"Atowe injowe! Atowe injowe!" Lillian could not understand what Kacha wanted.

"Give her your nail file." Mami said.

Then with the file in her left hand Kacha was trying to cut the apple!

The next stage after this, when she wanted something was:

"Awa! "Awa! = "There you are" "There you are". This reasoning came out when she was allowed to have something, the statement "There you are" was made when handing it over to her.

Among babies -

Whenever Kacha is with another baby or among other babies, they were all chattering together in their baby language.

Brrr, aah, waay, hee hee, eee...and real laughter!

Semba -

From age two months Kacha Walo was put on a pink potty on Mami's lap. She soon realised that the potty was the proper place to do it.

She first caught the phrase 'chamber pot', but only the beginning of the phrase: 'semba' which stuck in her mind.

Whenever she wanted to answer the call of nature, she would say:

"Semba! Semba!."

Sometimes she would crawl towards the semba in the bedroom and pick it up but to remove her nappy was beyond her.

Babati -

Nappy-changing was a great battle. Kacha hated it. To make her interested, while lightly smacking her bottom with talcum powder on her hand, Mami says:

"Powder! Pha! Pha! Pha!"

There ended the hate of nappy-changing, it became simplified, as Kacha Walo was looking forward to nappy-changing, so she could sing:

"Babati! Pa! Pa! Pa! Babati Pa! Pa! Pa!"

Chatter of the pub -

Kacha Walo's Papa (grand dad) tells her about the men in the pub, and how they talked in their merry-making.

Gidi is not only the pram pusher who took much pleasure in pushing the pram, sometimes at high speed, while Kacha loudly imitated the sound of a motor car, but he was also the listener to Kacha's stories in her mimic language. With all her might while dancing about on her bottom (she could not stand yet!), she would say:

Ayu! Wayu! Wayu! - Ayu! Wayu! Wayu! The pub chatter!

Buci. Buci -

They were in the dining room.   Mami was engaged in something at the dining table. At six months old, Kacha was sitting in the pram and Fido the cat was on the side of the pram.

Kacha overreached to touch Fido, and over balanced, tripped out of the pram and fell to the ground. It was a scary moment for all. She cried calling:

"Buci! Buci!" Pussy! Pussy!

Then there was a time from age four months when Kacha did not want to eat her breakfast porridge. She shook her head and blew the teaspoon-full porridge out of her mouth. So, Mami brought toys on the table to help with the feeding. When Kacha was busy with some toy, mother put in her mouth a spoon of porridge. She would, subconsciously, take a couple of spoons but once she realised she was eating, she blew it out! What would have taken half an hour to accomplish took longer, with the toy games in between.

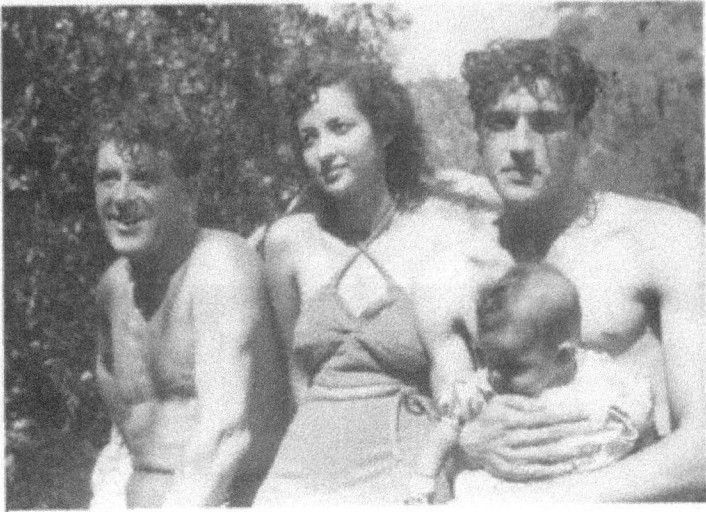

At five months with Dad (Francis right), Mami and friend Eric

Likabula natural swimming pools, Mulanje

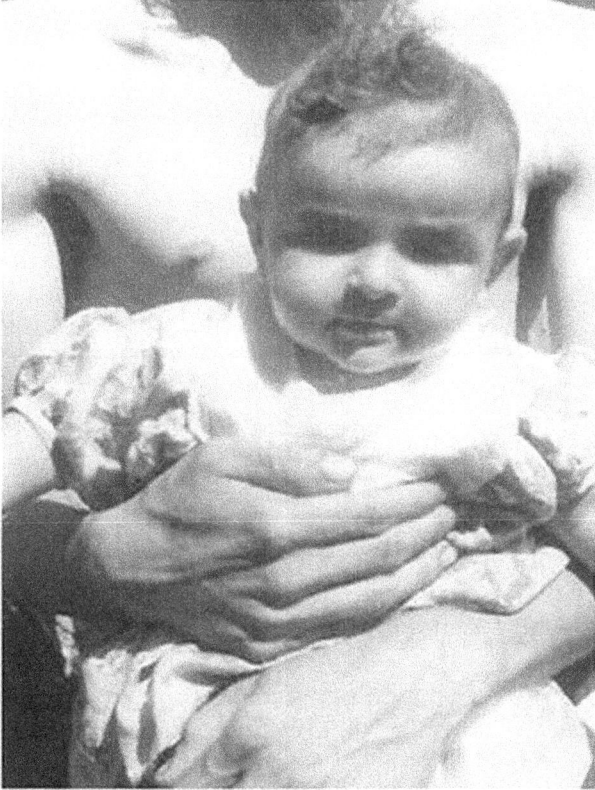

Lorna and Dad

At ten months Kacha began to crawl. The best crawling area was Granny's house which had a long passage flanked by four bedrooms and two bathrooms on either side.

She had a little song to go with the crawling:

"E..ee...ee"

She wore a little gold bangle on each wrist and the bangles clicked on the polished floor, as she went:

"E..ee...ee – ting (the bangles) "

"E..ee...ee – ting...

"E..ee...ee – ting...

****

Then came the time of balloons. Kacha, like most children was terribly excited about balloons.

One night in her sleep, while in dreamland, she shouted:

"Baalooniee!"

At the time Mami was working for R H Kirkcaldy and she told this dream of balloon to her boss, Mrs Kirkcaldy who gave her one shilling to buy some balloons for Lorna. In those days it was one penny for one balloon. Kacha was overwhelmed with twelve balloons.

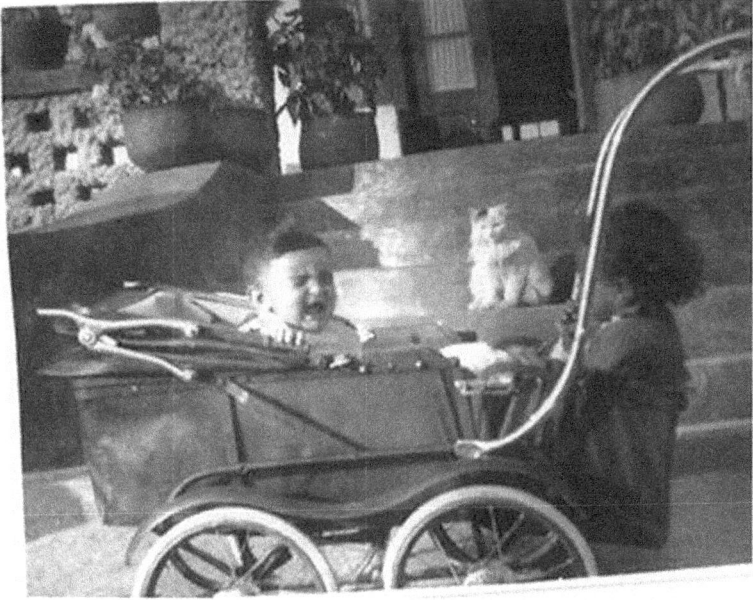

Kacha and Bina having a fight in the pram, with Fido the cat, as referee

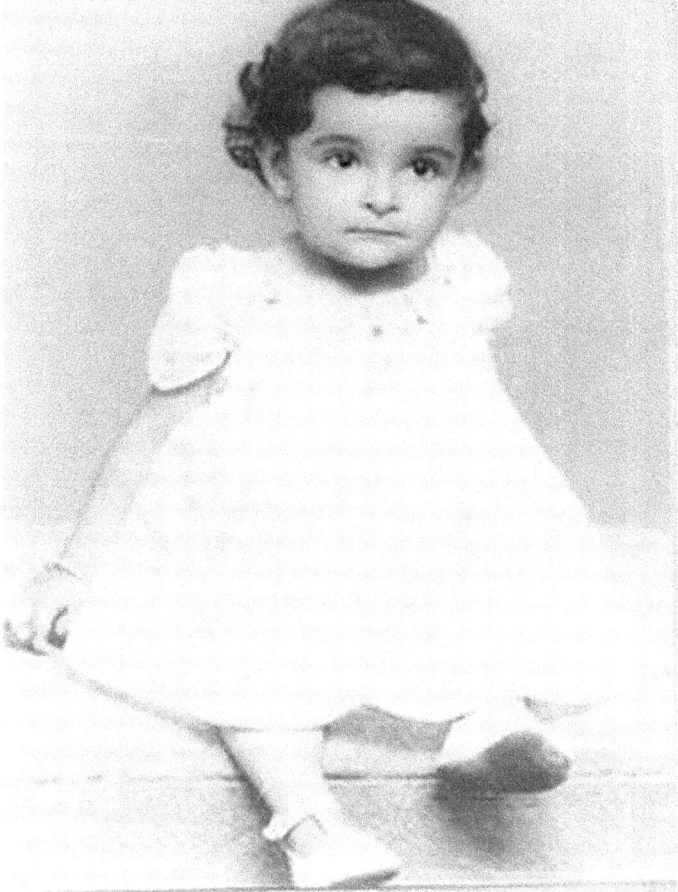

Kacha at fifteen months

Kacha at fifteen months did not want her picture taken. We were at the Blantyre Studio. Nanda, Mami's friend decided to make funny signs with her hands and facial movements, then that attracted the poser momentarily when the camera clicked!

We went for a walk with Kacha in her pram. As we reached the main road there was a 7-ton lorry loaded with firewood. The lorry assistant was sitting on the top of the firewood.

Kacha looked up and said:

"Eee – wagatu" – agwa (Chichewa) meaning he will fall off!

When she fell herself she would say:

"Waga". [She] Has fallen.

This was the stage of the 'third' person speech most babies go through. Otherwise in the first person speech it would be "Ndagwa", I have fallen in Chichewa.

****

2

FIRST BIRTHDAY ANNIVERSAY

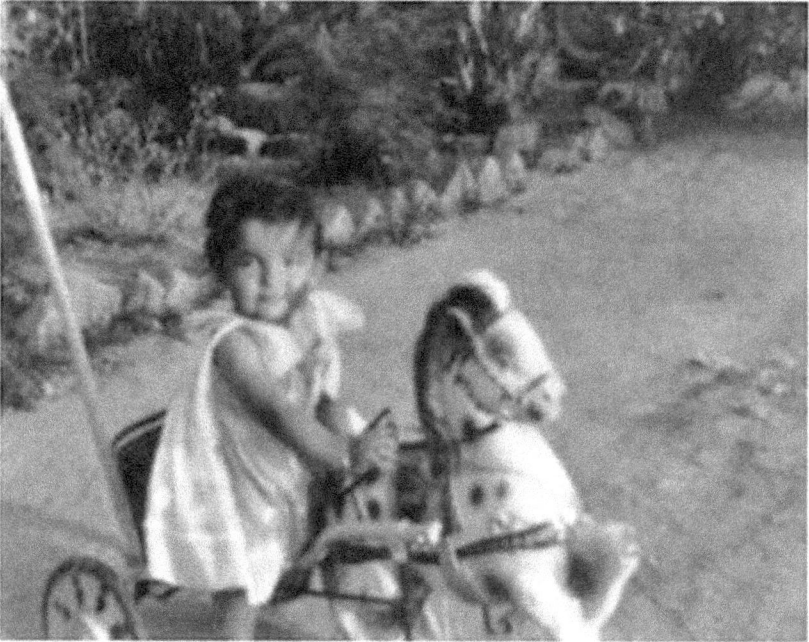

Kacha on her horse

Her daddy sent her a toy horse.

Wosey! Wosey! -

Kacha sitting on her little dapple grey horse, saying:

"Wosey! Wosey! Lookoo sani"

Horsey" Horsey! Look at the sun!

Kacha's first birthday party - was a great event for her. She was all awareness and knowing that some great event about herself was taking place. She received many messages of congratulations.

A message from the Baileys:

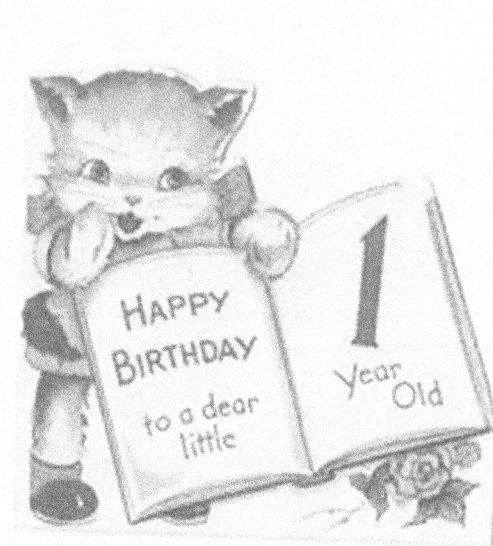

To Lorna, dear little one for whom life has just began. There are plenty of stories untold for the girl who is one year old!! And, so, we'll all give one big cheer, for you, little Lorna, dear. With all our love: Elizabeth, Catherine, John, Uncle Eric and Aunty Shula – pronounced as 'Aunt Cula' by Kacha.

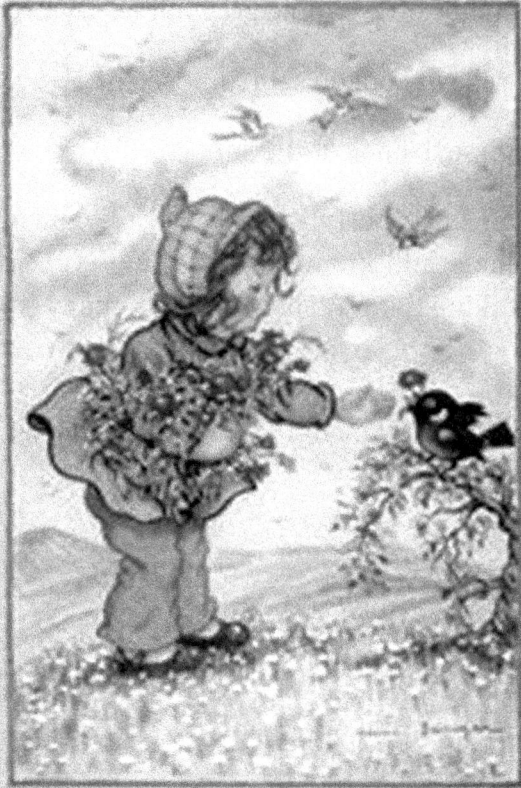

To wish you Happy Birthday

From Dr Antao and family

Kacha ate a whole samosa and the party went one till she slumped into a deep sleep – 09:00 pm! She was carried to bed. Since she was born she was up at 5:00 am, not a minute late or early.

On the morning after this grand occasion she was late waking up, 6:30 am, from the party hangover!. She was covered in mosh, phoo! Mami never saw so much mosh from a little baby – it must have been the samosa...

The word 'mosh' (motion) was formed by the little ones, Lorna and Bina, to mean excrement (or faeces, waste matter discharged from the bowels), a term the adults adopted (among others!).

Teece bada!

Kacha Walo had realised that teething powder wrapped up in white paper from the chemist gave her relief. Whenever she was in pain, during teething she called:

"Teece bada! Teece bada!"

"Teething powder!" "Teething powder!"

Pasina -

Vaseline she pronounced as 'pasina', the popular brand of petroleum jelly good for baby's bottom.

Then came the stage where almost everything to Kacha was 'dati' as she became 'dirt' conscious. She struggled to remove Mami's mole on her upper lip saying:

"Dati!" Dati" "Dirty" "Dirty!"

While stretching her hands constantly she would demand:

"Washansi!" "Washansi!" "Wash hands!" "Wash hands!"

Kacha was shown a picture of her Mami at age 18 months, and explained to her that was her Mami. Kacha got that confused look on her face, she could not connect her mother as a baby..

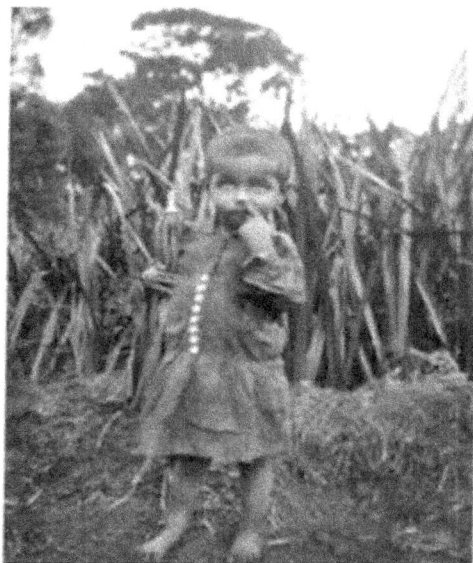

"Mami?" Kacha asked

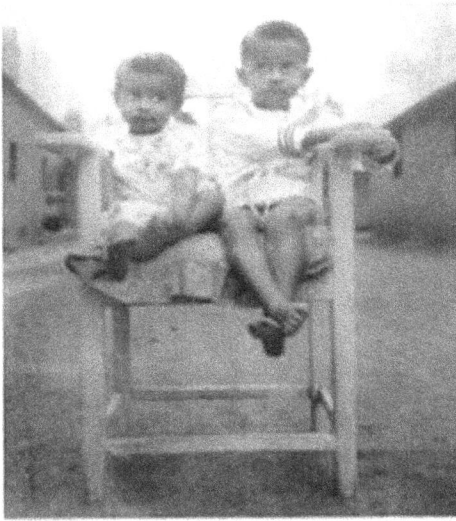

Mami (Rose) and brother Cader 1932

When Kacha was eighteen months, on 6th May 1954, her baby brother Joseph was born. When he was a few hours old Granny had him on her lap. Kacha came along and said

"Odi!" - meaning "Excuse me" in ChiChewa.

Then the midwife took the baby and Kacha sat on Granny's lap with the 'contented' look on her face as if to say "this is 'my' rightful place."

Joseph was a 'blue' baby, the cord was round his neck when he was born. Sadly, he did not make it and passed on four days later.

3

ON CLOTHING:

Shuta -

Whenever Kacha saw someone wearing a sweater, cardigan or any knitted garment, she would say:

"Shuta!". Sweater. She had grasped the descriptive name of the first knitted garment she came across.

Cusi – Not only the shoes she was wearing or what shoes she wanted to wear, but liked to point at other people's shoes:

"Cusi. Cusi".

Deshi -

She would point out the dress she wanted to wear by repeating:

"Deshi! Deshi!"

Ati -

She sees a hat or someone wearing a hat or asking to wear her hat, she would say:

"Ati! Ati!"

On Edibles

Maney – Chimanga (chiChewa).

Green boiled maize (or sweet corn as the Americans say).

This later developed to 'mandey'.

Kaku = Guava

Tutsi = Sweets

Colocate = Chocolate

Lolobes = Strawberries

Manana = Banana

On other things -

Ayusi -

When she sees a house anywhere or she is in the pram after an outing calling for homeward bound:

"Ayusi! Ayusi!" "House!" "House!"

Moo -

Moo! Moo!" When she sees Cows in the field.

Lala -

Eh! Lala!" "Eh! Fire!"

Chair -

Kacha did not catch the word 'chair', instead when she saw a chair she used a whole sentence:

"Tidani!" "Tidani!" "Sit down!" "Sit down!"

Telling that the item was for 'sitting' down.

When something upset Kacha Walo she cried, screaming on top of her voice:"

"Poo bebe Kasha!" "Poor baby Kacha!!"

"Poo Walo!" "Poor Walo!"

****

We often visited the Baileys and on one occasion there was another female guest there. They began to talk about Lorna (Kacha) on who she looked like, discussing her features, like her mother or father?

All the women said she looked like her father and there was nothing of her mother in her.

Eric said;

"What are you saying, she is a 'girl', isn't she!?"

****

Kacha was not upset, she was quietly observing all around her and the statement that followed put everyone in their place, and all were surprised that Kacha was capable of forming a meaningful sentence.

She politely but firmly uttered only three words:

"Leave Lona alone!"

Another of Kacha's little unexpected outbursts when she was only six months old Mami was cleaning her nose and she was resisting, as a result of which it caused her nose to bleed.

Then one day totally unexpected she shoved her little finger into Mami's nose and caused it to bleed. Kacha had a satisfied smug look and smile on her face. A kind of 'tit for tat' as it were!

Mami did her deep breathing exercises at night just after Kacha had fallen asleep. On one occasion she was not quite asleep so she asked what Mami was doing and she was told that Mami was doing her daily deep breathing exercises. The next day before she fell asleep, she was breathing heavily. Mami asked:

"What are you doing?"

"Breevin". Kacha replied.

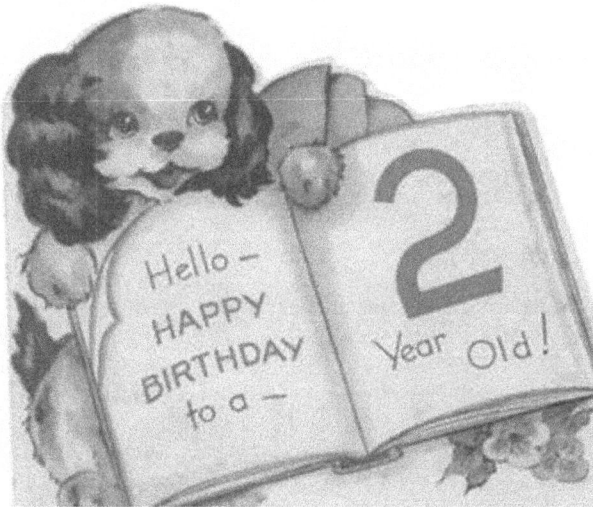

Alole was one of two little girls who were taken from their home in Mangochi by Kacha's grand parents at the girls' request to come to Blantyre and earn some cash. The other girl was looking after Bina. It was a temporary arrangement to mind the little ones, Bina and Lorna. The girls retuned to Mangochi after earning the cash they needed – brave little girls.

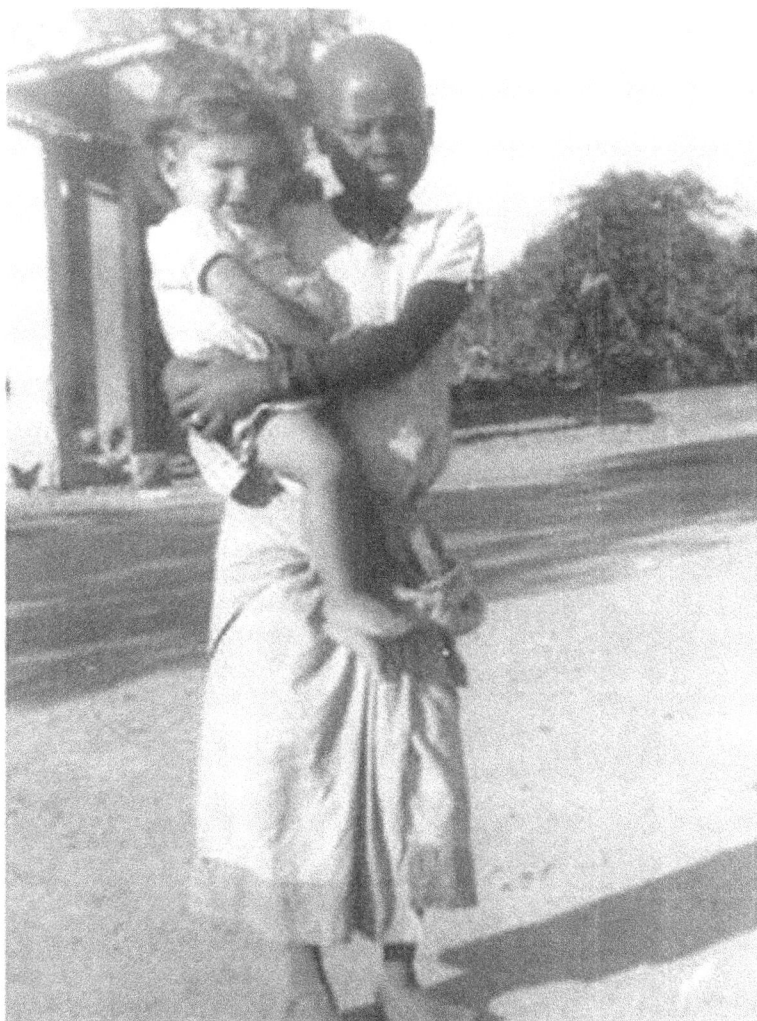

Kacha at two with Alole

When Kacha was two and a half years old Mami was to make the most difficult decision: to study a secretarial course at Pitman's College, London and leave behind little Kacha with her Ganni and Papa .

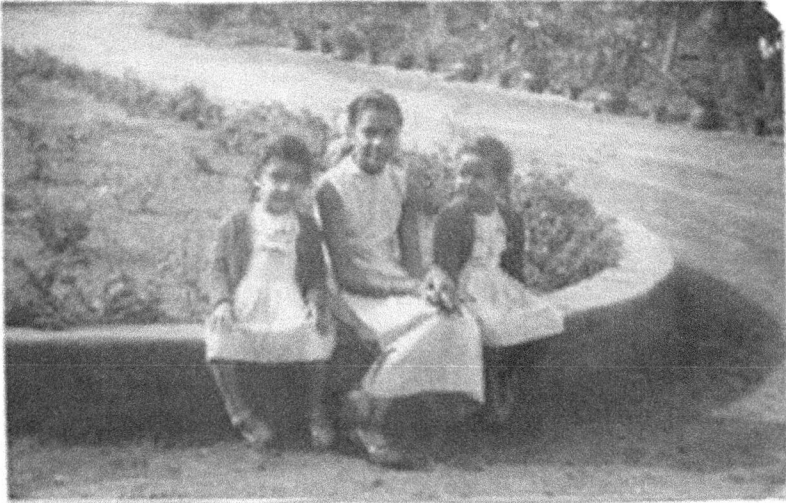

Picture taken by Ganni in her beautiful garden

Kacha (left) with Ellen and Bina

Shulayuzi -

Kacha loved and praised flowers. When she saw flowers she would say: "Eeh shulayuzi!"

One day Mami carrying Kacha they was walking in Ganni's beautiful garden when Kacha wanted to touch a rose bush.

Mami said:

"Don't touch roses, they have naughty thorns."

That puzzled look came on Kacha's face. She pointed a finger at Mami (Rose) and said:

"This one noti?" ("This one naughty?")

She could not visualise her Mami (Rose) as 'naughty'.

****

From about the age of four Kacha's weapon of censure was:

"I am going to the bush to find lion. He will eat me up and you shall never see this face of mine again!"

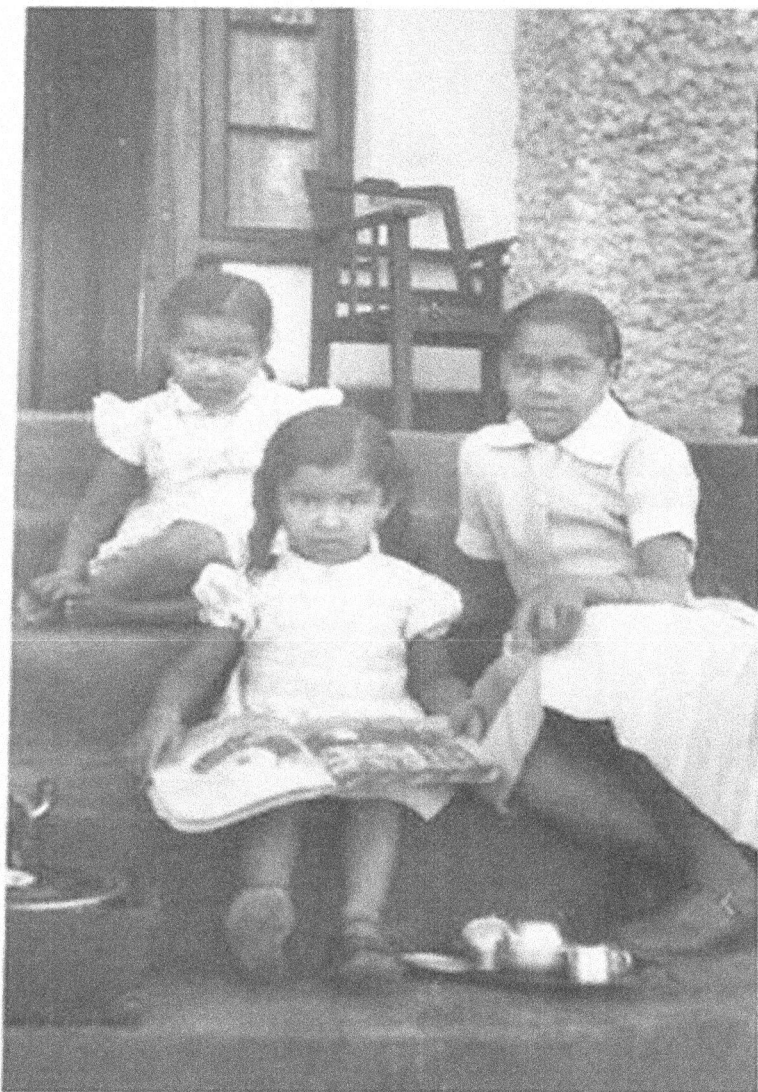

Kacha on her third birthday with Ellen and Bina

Mami sent her a record singing "Happy Birthday" recorded in a London music studio to the accompanyment of a piano (left on the picture, barely visible, playing on the gramophone of that time, "His Master's Voice", see *Caesar and Mapanga*

Homestead).

Kacha' Auntie Yvonne liked to tickle her. Protesting Kacha would say in Chichewa;

"Eee! Baci!" Meaning 'basi' enough!

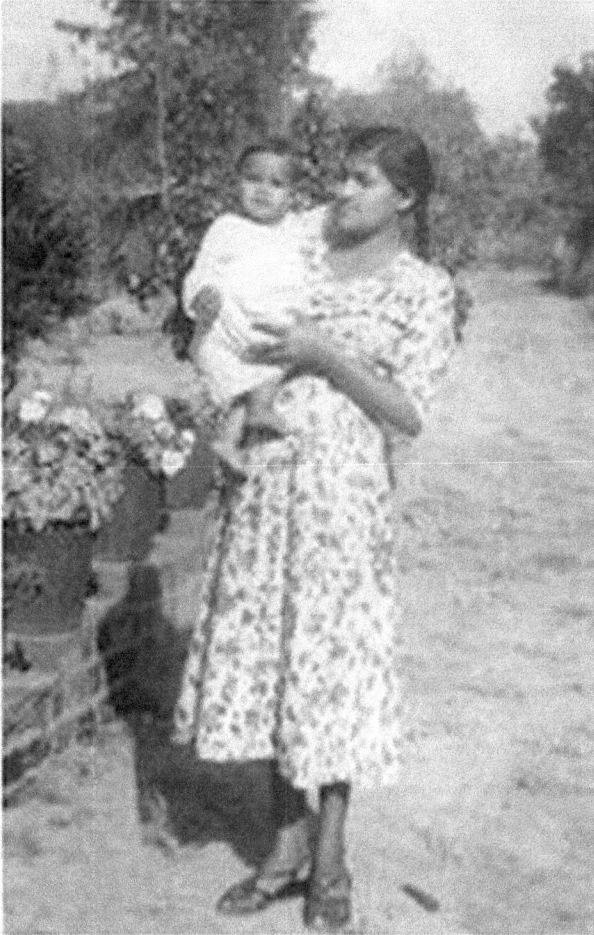

David with mother Yvonne - the youngest grand child

of Hannah and Joseph before the birth of Roxanne

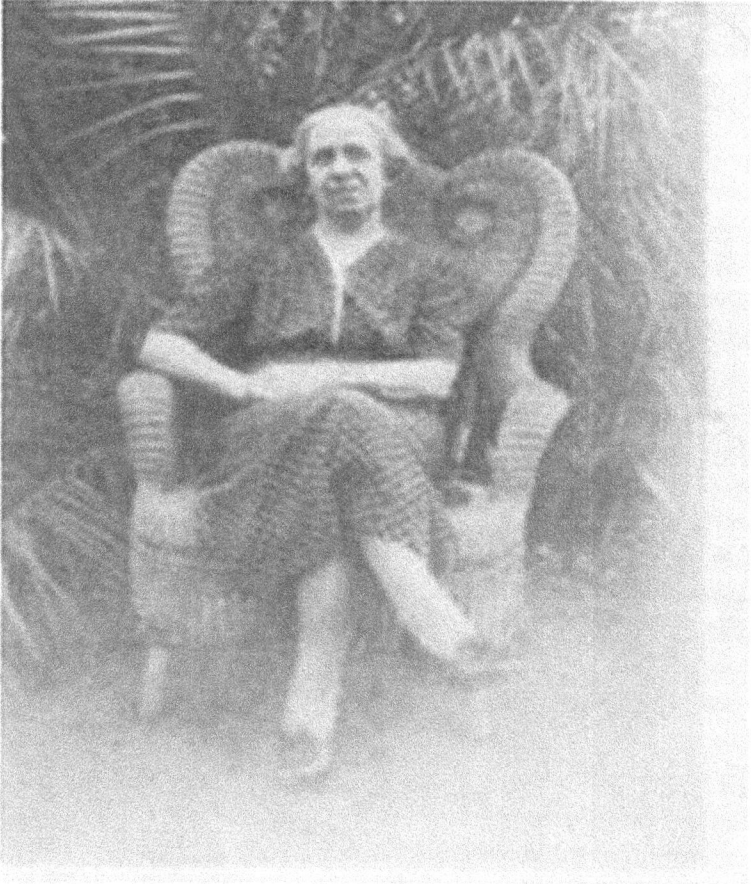

Emma Louiza Argente

Kacha's great grand mother

Emma Louiza was born in Portugal and lived in Lourenco Marques, Portuguese East Africa (now Maputo, Mozambique), with her husband Honor Argente. He was French and a shipper in Lourenco Marques.

****

EPILOGUE -

How do we come into being?

Embryoblast is the beginning of every human, a combination of Eve's Cell and Adam's sperm. Heterosexual union generates life through gene containing chromosomes found in the nucleus of a cell. The cell is basic to all forms of life, plants, animals, and humans. The human body contains billions of cells, or building units, which are replaced every seven years during one's lifespan. All parts of the human body, blood, skin, muscle, nerve, bone and tissue are made up of different cells which relate to their particular functions. This is apparent in medical treatment: each part of our anatomy is treated by a different and particular kind of medicine when those cells fail. The process of heredity is essentially similar in all species of life. Physiological processes operate to produce and distribute variation and enables natural selection to function. Cellular characteristics, genes, chromosomes and DNA are found in the cells of all plants, animals, and humans.

Two kinds of cells are directly involved with heredity, somatic cells and sex cells. Somatic cells, the structural composition of the body, divide by *mitosis,* which produces two daughter cells identical to each other and to the mother cell. Sex cells divide twice by *meiosis*, and produce four gametes; and they originate in the testes of males and ovaries of females, whose function is to transmit life and hereditary information from parents to progeny. From head to toe, human sperm cells measure about 50 micrometers (0.05 millimetre, or roughly 0.002 inch). The tiniest object you can see with your unaided eyes is about 0.1 mm – so forget about seeing sperm without a microscope. A human egg is about 30 times bigger, large enough to be seen with the naked eye.

A cell consists of two parts, nucleus or focal point, and cytoplasm, the parts which are not the nucleus. These invisible, spherical billions of cells in the human body are like chambers or units in which chromosomes are confined. Chromosomes are hereditary messages, which determine characteristics. They are threadlike, gene-containing, found in the nucleus of a cell. They come in pairs because they were inherited in pairs, and would be inherited in pairs, and passed from generation to generation in a blending theory. Since each of the female and male reproduction cells contain 46 chromosomes one would expect the new cell to have 92 chromosomes, but meiosis is a self-halving process.

This is what happens:

    46 diploid number chromosomes

       of the sperm cell halve themselves

       to haploid number .... .23) they combine

    46 diploid number chromosomes of) to make a new

       of the egg cell halve themselves) cell, zygote,

       haploid number...................23) which carries

                   46 chromosomes.

  Sex determination of offspring:

      22 autosomes from father   )

      1 sex chromosome either   ) = 23 pairs of

        X = female   )

heterogeneous

        Y = male   ) chromosomes.

The process of halving is not by random collection of any 23 chromosomes, but of gametes, which when combined with the other sex cell can form a fertilised cell, containing reproductive value. The zygote, consists of an organism of fifty per cent from each parent but is *unique*, identical to neither parent. No two people are alike (except identical twins). Take a billion people and you have a billion varieties and this makes selection possible. Each chromosome bears 2000 smaller particles, complex chemical chains, the genes, structured in a double helix ladder with a vertical twist of deoxyribonucleic acid, DNA, and all information is stored in molecules of this substance. Sometimes two ova may shed simultaneously from the ovary and each of them may be fertilised and develop normally. The consequence of this is the *dizygote,* fraternal twins, with an independent genetic constitution, they may be male and female, both male, or both female. Twins can also arise from a single fertilised ovum, *monozygote*, identical twins. *Zygotes* and *dizygotes* have unique DNA. *Monozygotes* share the same DNA. In some instances identical cells may separate themselves into two or more organisms and lead to identical twins, triplets, or more. The left handed person had a mirror twin in the womb and the other simply disintegrated into the debris of the womb.

Genes function in pairs to influence hereditary characteristics from each parent. The individual members of pairs of genes are the alleles, or one or two alternative forms of gene. The alleles regulate the occurrence of certain discrete proportions, such as colour of eyes, colour of hair, and other characteristic traits. The dominant alleles influence is expressed in some pairs and the non-dominant is said to be recessive. Lack of the production of a critical enzyme in genes influences the overproduction of phenylypyruvic acid, which causes the disease of phynyketonuria of genetic defects and which may lead to mental retardation and other disorders. There is the possibility that in the year 2050 by advanced research and development of the subject a sub-microscopic piece of DNA may afford an extra gene inserted in every cell of the female body to give the recipient a lifelong resistance against the virus that causes AIDS.

Individual generic make up is determined at conception. Other circumstances are also influencing factors, such as *recombination, mutation, genetic drift*, and *migration.* In any sexually reproducing species both parents contribute genes to offspring in recombination and genetic information is reshuffled every generation and reshuffling would not cause evolution. Mutation is an alteration of genetic material, a molecular alteration. If mutation does not take place in the sperm or ovum it will not pass to the next generation and evolution will not occur. Genetic drift is caused by a number of factors, which act on the size of the population and size of group. Where individual or individuals are reduced either by death or migration the genes would have been removed from the population of the group. Then evolution would occur, upon which natural selection acts, the process of favouring survival or organisms best adapted to their environment. A trait must be inherited to have importance in natural selection, in evolution, and variation in inherited characteristic. Migration occurs where people migrate and mate in groups different from their own, and gene frequency would be altered.

The changes in gene content that may occur through recombination, mutation, recombination, genetic drift, or migration do not alter the characteristic of the beginning of every individual as a microscopic dot. The transmission of female or male genitalia in the naturals depends on chromosomal dominance and in the un-naturals would depend on the choice of parent or parents.

The female ovaries, two almond-shaped organs measuring about one and one half inch long lie in the area between the vagina and navel, the channel to the womb. The ovaries produce female hormones which stimulate energy and dynamism, the pep in female, and trigger physiological changes such as breast development at puberty, the pre-nubile stage. The hormones also mobilise the ovaries' ova, the eggs, which fertilise when penetrated by sperm. Leading from the ovaries are the Fallopian tubes, two thin ducts, which meet at the pear-shaped womb. Female external organs, the labia majora, covered with hair, are two folds of tissues, which resemble lips, enclose the genitals. Internally, and underneath the labia majora is another pair of lips, labia minora, an intricate elegant clitoral system that extends deep inside the female genitals and fills with blood the basis of intense feelings of pleasure and contain oil and sweat glands. At the tip buried in muscle and fibrous tissue, is a small bud of tissue, the clitoris, the most sensitive organ of the female anatomy. The labia are the gate to the vagina and the channel to the womb. The clitoris with introverted genitals, as David Niven puts it is "a flat arrangement" (*The Moon is a Balloon*), seemingly less aggressive than male extroverted genitalia. The clitoris is descended from the same embryonic structure that becomes the male penis when the Y sex chromosome dominates.

In the male, the urinary track lies at the bottom of the bladder beside the prostrate gland. The urethra passes along the penis and enables muscles at the base to exude urine through a minute opening at the lip of the corona. The lip of the penis is acon-shaped and separate from the shaft by a rim of tissue, the corona or crown at birth is covered by foreskin. In the female, the bladder lies above the uterus and vagina. The urethra exits the body in front of the vagina, within the labia folds. Of all primates, only man does not have a penile bone. His upright stature and bipedal motion expose the penis to danger. Most primates spend their lives hanging or brachiating in branches. In many animals the female has the equivalent of penile bone. Cats, seals and rodents, and many others have both penile and clitoral bones.

The puberty stage for the female is between nine and thirteen years and for the male ten to fifteen years. In the female, the ovaries secrete female hormones, oestrogen and progesterone.

These cause breasts to develop, the hips to broaden, and pubic and underarms hair to appear, menstruation begins about the same time. In the male, the testes secrete the male hormone testosterone, which triggers the growth of facial, body and pubic hair, an increase is muscle bulk, a deepening of the voice, growth of the genital organs and the development of sperm in the testes However, at puberty the increase in testosterone is huge and so causes the development of testes at puberty; and female individuals may become male at puberty, the. Very rarely this may not work and children are born as female but genetically male. They are insensitive to androgens, male hormones. The Androgen Insensitive Syndrome may be the influencing factor in homosexuality tendencies.

The female glands are heated in coitus stimulated fluid and the clitoris, like the penis, swells with blood during sexual arousal. Only in a few women does the clitoris become fully erect. The labia accommodates the penis and conveys the sperm cell from father to mother's left oviduct. A single male ejaculation exudes enough sperm to fertilise and populate an entire continent but only less than one per cent of the spermatozoon are the fertile ovum-getters. More than one spermatozoon may, simultaneously, race to the fertilisation point – sperm awareness in its sojourn from the start of the race. The spermatozoa has a lashing tail, tips empowered by chromosome energy, void of limbs, but agile, and is an accomplished swimmer. Sperm writhes on the surface of the ovum which draws them to it. Although only one spermatozoa, embryoblast, will gain entry to the ovum and fertilise it, a good number of spermatozoon break down the ovum cell's outer coating by releasing protein-dissolving enzymes before the embryoblast can gain entry. Besides the labours of fellow candidates to break the outer coating and the magnetism of the ovum to draw sperm to it, two factors aid the winner: determination to outrace fellow candidates (when unruly offspring confront parents and say "I did not beg to be born", it is not entirely true) and head small enough to penetrate the ovum, Once through the gate, the ovum will close its barriers and the rest of the contestants expire infantile sperm and from the moment of conception the winner is *mortal*. Fusion of the nucleus of the sperm head and that of the ovum, a microscopic dot, produces the *zygot. Every zygote is female at conception.* From the moment of conception the zygote is incubated in the mother's womb for nine months, oblivious to and unaware of external surroundings and travels through a route of development.

The embryoblast has three phases of development, the *zygote*, the *embryo*, and the *foetus*. The zygote phase is two weeks from conception. Rapid development of the zygote into an embryo occurs mainly within the lining of the uterus but it actually begins while the ovum is travelling down the fallopian tube by concentration of energy and divides into diploid number of cells: $1 + 1 = 2$; $2 + 2 = 4$; $4 + 4 = 8$, and so on, to form the embryo. In addition the embryoblast produces trophoblast cells that develop into the placenta, a gauze of membrane of the womb which enwraps the zygote to supply oxygen and nutrients to the baby from its mother through the umbilical cord and carry away waste product. The environment of each cell is the cytoplasm, the living substance surrounding the cell nucleus. The placenta, and the umbilical cord develop to link indirectly the bloodstream of the embryo to the mother's separated by cell walls. Both bloodstreams pass into the placenta, semi-permeable membranes prevent passage of blood cells but allows nutrients from mother's blood to escape through to embryo and waste from embryo to mother. In the nine-month of unified existence the embryo becomes a *receiving station within a receiving station*. Therefore, the mother's possible intake of unsuitable diet, such as nicotine, alcohol, or infected semen may cause adverse effects or the consequences of sexually transmitted diseases (with the rife of AIDS a great number of infants throughout the world have been infected with the virus contacted within the womb via mother's bloodstream) over which an embryo has no control. From the embryo the foetus unfolds.

The marked characteristic of the foetus from eight weeks to forty weeks of conception is rapid progression of intricate structures of sensory cells, blood cells, nerve cells and other cells that form the human frame. Mother's womb expands to accommodate the progressing foetus and cells are active with purpose to the endurance of the entire foetus. Floating, heeding intrinsic commands, oblivious to but faintly aware of latent sounds and surroundings; invisible, yet evident, metaphor of posterity, the minute absolute monarch of the bubble within travels for nine months its allocation of lineal time.

Sex is genetically determined at fertilisation and all embryos develop as female until the genes from the Y chromosome 'kick in' at the time of genital development. Very rarely and mysteriously the *mould shakes* when there is a case of ambiguous genitalia in newborns. Either due to a developmental physical defect or due to a lack of, or too much of, certain hormones, for some inexplicable reasons the testes appear on one side of the midline and an ovary on the other side and produce both male and female ducts. The result is a hermaphrodite, sexually abnormal individual, seen by other societies as a bad omen and the baby is destroyed.

XY has a fifty-fifty chance of carrying an X and an equal chance of carrying a Y. Three weeks after fertilisation gonads, sex glands, will form on either side of the midline of the reptilian shaped embryo. At this stage sex glands have been programmed by the parent sex chromosomes. The Y chromosome causes formation of the Wolfaan (male) duct system and the rest of the anatomy will develop as male. The embryonic testes in addition produce anti-Mullerian (anti-female) duct system, important in sexual features. In the XX individuals the gonads will become ovaries and will produce large quantities of oestrogen and lesser quantities of testosterone. Given the muliebrity state of the embryo that is why men have female features such as nipples and mammary glands. The interaction of genes and uterine environmental conditions produce physical traits, a feature that could also enhance homosexuality, a sexual trait still seen as taboo in certain societies but has been gradually tolerated, yet to be accepted, in Western societies.

At 28 months baby is fully formed but has three more stages before delivery. The amnionic sac around the baby raptures and fluid drains away. Muscles of mother's womb then begin to contract and the neck of the cervix dilates, may take up to ten hours and contractions occur more frequently. Baby moves down the birth canal, in a normal birth, head emerges first, may take two hours for first baby. In a breach situation baby is born feet or buttocks first having failed to turn during pregnancy. Before 37 weeks of pregnancy baby may be born prematurely, or if mother and baby are at risk baby may be born through caesarean section, and sometimes a fully formed baby at 38 weeks is stillborn (dies in the womb before birth). After birth the placenta is expelled. Hormone release during the birth triggers mother's breasts to produce colostrums, a rich precursor to milk. Some great men such as Socranus, of Euphesus, Greece, in the fifteenth century CE advocated literacy for the midwife in order that she understood the importance of baby's safe delivery in comforting the labouring mother.

On the day of birth father (if there is one), is a wreck of worry. Baby exudes helpless, handicapped, no limb to touch, or bipedal, gasping for air, no speech to communicate and enters the world *yelling*. Pain from the sudden egress, anger and fright at separation from the protection of the womb or charged with like velocity to the fertilising point at conception? Nonetheless, baby's first cry is a sweet melody to present ears. Now he or she is a *receiving station* for parental nurture and social conditioning.

The start of our journey through life carries no strategies to enable us to cope with the mental, emotional and spiritual aspects but then life is a journey of discovery. Society with all its philosophers and diverse mentors has regarded the individual as lacking the innate capacity to classify our world over the centuries; sees itself as the prescription of the role model for the individual. Life begins in the confinement of a cell through stages to the second stage of another cell from the moment of birth, a fragile, transparent cell through life. From it is the individual's image of the world as conditioned to see it.

A pictorial passage about Kacha Walo (nicknamed by Granny), on her journey of discovery; how she learns by mimicking what is happening around her; how she picks up words in her own baby language, converses with other babies in their own baby language; and her vocabulary influences adults as a more subtle way to express oneself; and how she views adult actions.

www.ingramcontent.com/pod-product-compliance
Lightning Source LLC
Chambersburg PA
CBHW071141280326

41935CB00010B/1315